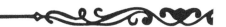

BLOOD SUGAR LOG BOOK

Personal Data

Name: _____

Phone: _____

Address: _____

Notes: _____

Emergency Contact

Name: _____

Phone: _____

Address: _____

Notes: _____

Doctor's Contact Information

Doctor: _____

Pharmacy: _____

Eye Clinic: _____

Dentist: _____

Notes: _____

Weekly Blood Sugar Log

Week: _____   Weight: _____

Day	Meal	Before	After	Notes
Monday > > >	Breakfast			
	Lunch			
	Dinner			
	Bedtime			

Day	Meal	Before	After	Notes
Tuesday > > >	Breakfast			
	Lunch			
	Dinner			
	Bedtime			

Day	Meal	Before	After	Notes
Wednesday > > >	Breakfast			
	Lunch			
	Dinner			
	Bedtime			

Day	Meal	Before	After	Notes
Thursday > > >	Breakfast			
	Lunch			
	Dinner			
	Bedtime			

Day	Meal	Before	After	Notes
Friday > > >	Breakfast			
	Lunch			
	Dinner			
	Bedtime			

Day	Meal	Before	After	Notes
Saturday > > >	Breakfast			
	Lunch			
	Dinner			
	Bedtime			

Day	Meal	Before	After	Notes
Sunday > > >	Breakfast			
	Lunch			
	Dinner			
	Bedtime			

Weekly Blood Sugar Log

Week: _____   Weight: _____

Day	Meal	Before	After	Notes
Monday > > >	Breakfast			
	Lunch			
	Dinner			
	Bedtime			

Day	Meal	Before	After	Notes
Tuesday > > >	Breakfast			
	Lunch			
	Dinner			
	Bedtime			

Day	Meal	Before	After	Notes
Wednesday > > >	Breakfast			
	Lunch			
	Dinner			
	Bedtime			

Day	Meal	Before	After	Notes
Thursday > > >	Breakfast			
	Lunch			
	Dinner			
	Bedtime			

Day	Meal	Before	After	Notes
Friday > > >	Breakfast			
	Lunch			
	Dinner			
	Bedtime			

Day	Meal	Before	After	Notes
Saturday > > >	Breakfast			
	Lunch			
	Dinner			
	Bedtime			

Day	Meal	Before	After	Notes
Sunday > > >	Breakfast			
	Lunch			
	Dinner			
	Bedtime			

Weekly Blood Sugar Log

Week: _____   Weight: _____

Day	Meal	Before	After	Notes
Monday > > >	Breakfast			
	Lunch			
	Dinner			
	Bedtime			

Day	Meal	Before	After	Notes
Tuesday > > >	Breakfast			
	Lunch			
	Dinner			
	Bedtime			

Day	Meal	Before	After	Notes
Wednesday > > >	Breakfast			
	Lunch			
	Dinner			
	Bedtime			

Day	Meal	Before	After	Notes
Thursday > > >	Breakfast			
	Lunch			
	Dinner			
	Bedtime			

Day	Meal	Before	After	Notes
Friday > > >	Breakfast			
	Lunch			
	Dinner			
	Bedtime			

Day	Meal	Before	After	Notes
Saturday > > >	Breakfast			
	Lunch			
	Dinner			
	Bedtime			

Day	Meal	Before	After	Notes
Sunday > > >	Breakfast			
	Lunch			
	Dinner			
	Bedtime			

Weekly Blood Sugar Log

Week: _____   Weight: _____

Day	Meal	Before	After	Notes
Monday > > >	Breakfast			
	Lunch			
	Dinner			
	Bedtime			

Day	Meal	Before	After	Notes
Tuesday > > >	Breakfast			
	Lunch			
	Dinner			
	Bedtime			

Day	Meal	Before	After	Notes
Wednesday > > >	Breakfast			
	Lunch			
	Dinner			
	Bedtime			

Day	Meal	Before	After	Notes
Thursday > > >	Breakfast			
	Lunch			
	Dinner			
	Bedtime			

Day	Meal	Before	After	Notes
Friday > > >	Breakfast			
	Lunch			
	Dinner			
	Bedtime			

Day	Meal	Before	After	Notes
Saturday > > >	Breakfast			
	Lunch			
	Dinner			
	Bedtime			

Day	Meal	Before	After	Notes
Sunday > > >	Breakfast			
	Lunch			
	Dinner			
	Bedtime			

Weekly Blood Sugar Log

Week: _____   Weight: _____

Day	Meal	Before	After	Notes
Monday > > >	Breakfast			
	Lunch			
	Dinner			
	Bedtime			

Day	Meal	Before	After	Notes
Tuesday > > >	Breakfast			
	Lunch			
	Dinner			
	Bedtime			

Day	Meal	Before	After	Notes
Wednesday > > >	Breakfast			
	Lunch			
	Dinner			
	Bedtime			

Day	Meal	Before	After	Notes
Thursday > > >	Breakfast			
	Lunch			
	Dinner			
	Bedtime			

Day	Meal	Before	After	Notes
Friday > > >	Breakfast			
	Lunch			
	Dinner			
	Bedtime			

Day	Meal	Before	After	Notes
Saturday > > >	Breakfast			
	Lunch			
	Dinner			
	Bedtime			

Day	Meal	Before	After	Notes
Sunday > > >	Breakfast			
	Lunch			
	Dinner			
	Bedtime			

Weekly Blood Sugar Log

Week: _____   Weight: _____

Day	Meal	Before	After	Notes
Monday > > >	Breakfast			
	Lunch			
	Dinner			
	Bedtime			

Day	Meal	Before	After	Notes
Tuesday > > >	Breakfast			
	Lunch			
	Dinner			
	Bedtime			

Day	Meal	Before	After	Notes
Wednesday > > >	Breakfast			
	Lunch			
	Dinner			
	Bedtime			

Day	Meal	Before	After	Notes
Thursday > > >	Breakfast			
	Lunch			
	Dinner			
	Bedtime			

Day	Meal	Before	After	Notes
Friday > > >	Breakfast			
	Lunch			
	Dinner			
	Bedtime			

Day	Meal	Before	After	Notes
Saturday > > >	Breakfast			
	Lunch			
	Dinner			
	Bedtime			

Day	Meal	Before	After	Notes
Sunday > > >	Breakfast			
	Lunch			
	Dinner			
	Bedtime			

Weekly Blood Sugar Log

Week: _____   Weight: _____

Day	Meal	Before	After	Notes
Monday > > >	Breakfast			
	Lunch			
	Dinner			
	Bedtime			

Day	Meal	Before	After	Notes
Tuesday > > >	Breakfast			
	Lunch			
	Dinner			
	Bedtime			

Day	Meal	Before	After	Notes
Wednesday > > >	Breakfast			
	Lunch			
	Dinner			
	Bedtime			

Day	Meal	Before	After	Notes
Thursday > > >	Breakfast			
	Lunch			
	Dinner			
	Bedtime			

Day	Meal	Before	After	Notes
Friday > > >	Breakfast			
	Lunch			
	Dinner			
	Bedtime			

Day	Meal	Before	After	Notes
Saturday > > >	Breakfast			
	Lunch			
	Dinner			
	Bedtime			

Day	Meal	Before	After	Notes
Sunday > > >	Breakfast			
	Lunch			
	Dinner			
	Bedtime			

Weekly Blood Sugar Log

Week: _____   Weight: _____

Day	Meal	Before	After	Notes
Monday > > >	Breakfast			
	Lunch			
	Dinner			
	Bedtime			

Day	Meal	Before	After	Notes
Tuesday > > >	Breakfast			
	Lunch			
	Dinner			
	Bedtime			

Day	Meal	Before	After	Notes
Wednesday > > >	Breakfast			
	Lunch			
	Dinner			
	Bedtime			

Day	Meal	Before	After	Notes
Thursday > > >	Breakfast			
	Lunch			
	Dinner			
	Bedtime			

Day	Meal	Before	After	Notes
Friday > > >	Breakfast			
	Lunch			
	Dinner			
	Bedtime			

Day	Meal	Before	After	Notes
Saturday > > >	Breakfast			
	Lunch			
	Dinner			
	Bedtime			

Day	Meal	Before	After	Notes
Sunday > > >	Breakfast			
	Lunch			
	Dinner			
	Bedtime			

Weekly Blood Sugar Log

Week: [blank]   Weight: [blank]

Day	Meal	Before	After	Notes
Monday > > >	Breakfast			
	Lunch			
	Dinner			
	Bedtime			

Day	Meal	Before	After	Notes
Tuesday > > >	Breakfast			
	Lunch			
	Dinner			
	Bedtime			

Day	Meal	Before	After	Notes
Wednesday > > >	Breakfast			
	Lunch			
	Dinner			
	Bedtime			

Day	Meal	Before	After	Notes
Thursday > > >	Breakfast			
	Lunch			
	Dinner			
	Bedtime			

Day	Meal	Before	After	Notes
Friday > > >	Breakfast			
	Lunch			
	Dinner			
	Bedtime			

Day	Meal	Before	After	Notes
Saturday > > >	Breakfast			
	Lunch			
	Dinner			
	Bedtime			

Day	Meal	Before	After	Notes
Sunday > > >	Breakfast			
	Lunch			
	Dinner			
	Bedtime			

Weekly Blood Sugar Log

Week: _____   Weight: _____

Day	Meal	Before	After	Notes
Monday > > >	Breakfast			
	Lunch			
	Dinner			
	Bedtime			

Day	Meal	Before	After	Notes
Tuesday > > >	Breakfast			
	Lunch			
	Dinner			
	Bedtime			

Day	Meal	Before	After	Notes
Wednesday > > >	Breakfast			
	Lunch			
	Dinner			
	Bedtime			

Day	Meal	Before	After	Notes
Thursday > > >	Breakfast			
	Lunch			
	Dinner			
	Bedtime			

Day	Meal	Before	After	Notes
Friday > > >	Breakfast			
	Lunch			
	Dinner			
	Bedtime			

Day	Meal	Before	After	Notes
Saturday > > >	Breakfast			
	Lunch			
	Dinner			
	Bedtime			

Day	Meal	Before	After	Notes
Sunday > > >	Breakfast			
	Lunch			
	Dinner			
	Bedtime			

Weekly Blood Sugar Log

Week: _____   Weight: _____

Day	Meal	Before	After	Notes
Monday > > >	Breakfast			
	Lunch			
	Dinner			
	Bedtime			

Day	Meal	Before	After	Notes
Tuesday > > >	Breakfast			
	Lunch			
	Dinner			
	Bedtime			

Day	Meal	Before	After	Notes
Wednesday > > >	Breakfast			
	Lunch			
	Dinner			
	Bedtime			

Day	Meal	Before	After	Notes
Thursday > > >	Breakfast			
	Lunch			
	Dinner			
	Bedtime			

Day	Meal	Before	After	Notes
Friday > > >	Breakfast			
	Lunch			
	Dinner			
	Bedtime			

Day	Meal	Before	After	Notes
Saturday > > >	Breakfast			
	Lunch			
	Dinner			
	Bedtime			

Day	Meal	Before	After	Notes
Sunday > > >	Breakfast			
	Lunch			
	Dinner			
	Bedtime			

Weekly Blood Sugar Log

Week: _____   Weight: _____

Day	Meal	Before	After	Notes
Monday > > >	Breakfast			
	Lunch			
	Dinner			
	Bedtime			

Day	Meal	Before	After	Notes
Tuesday > > >	Breakfast			
	Lunch			
	Dinner			
	Bedtime			

Day	Meal	Before	After	Notes
Wednesday > > >	Breakfast			
	Lunch			
	Dinner			
	Bedtime			

Day	Meal	Before	After	Notes
Thursday > > >	Breakfast			
	Lunch			
	Dinner			
	Bedtime			

Day	Meal	Before	After	Notes
Friday > > >	Breakfast			
	Lunch			
	Dinner			
	Bedtime			

Day	Meal	Before	After	Notes
Saturday > > >	Breakfast			
	Lunch			
	Dinner			
	Bedtime			

Day	Meal	Before	After	Notes
Sunday > > >	Breakfast			
	Lunch			
	Dinner			
	Bedtime			

Weekly Blood Sugar Log

Week: Weight:

Day	Meal	Before	After	Notes
Monday > > >	Breakfast			
	Lunch			
	Dinner			
	Bedtime			

Day	Meal	Before	After	Notes
Tuesday > > >	Breakfast			
	Lunch			
	Dinner			
	Bedtime			

Day	Meal	Before	After	Notes
Wednesday > > >	Breakfast			
	Lunch			
	Dinner			
	Bedtime			

Day	Meal	Before	After	Notes
Thursday > > >	Breakfast			
	Lunch			
	Dinner			
	Bedtime			

Day	Meal	Before	After	Notes
Friday > > >	Breakfast			
	Lunch			
	Dinner			
	Bedtime			

Day	Meal	Before	After	Notes
Saturday > > >	Breakfast			
	Lunch			
	Dinner			
	Bedtime			

Day	Meal	Before	After	Notes
Sunday > > >	Breakfast			
	Lunch			
	Dinner			
	Bedtime			

Weekly Blood Sugar Log

Week: _____   Weight: _____

Day	Meal	Before	After	Notes
Monday > > >	Breakfast			
	Lunch			
	Dinner			
	Bedtime			

Day	Meal	Before	After	Notes
Tuesday > > >	Breakfast			
	Lunch			
	Dinner			
	Bedtime			

Day	Meal	Before	After	Notes
Wednesday > > >	Breakfast			
	Lunch			
	Dinner			
	Bedtime			

Day	Meal	Before	After	Notes
Thursday > > >	Breakfast			
	Lunch			
	Dinner			
	Bedtime			

Day	Meal	Before	After	Notes
Friday > > >	Breakfast			
	Lunch			
	Dinner			
	Bedtime			

Day	Meal	Before	After	Notes
Saturday > > >	Breakfast			
	Lunch			
	Dinner			
	Bedtime			

Day	Meal	Before	After	Notes
Sunday > > >	Breakfast			
	Lunch			
	Dinner			
	Bedtime			

Weekly Blood Sugar Log

Week: _____   Weight: _____

Day	Meal	Before	After	Notes
Monday > > >	Breakfast			
	Lunch			
	Dinner			
	Bedtime			

Day	Meal	Before	After	Notes
Tuesday > > >	Breakfast			
	Lunch			
	Dinner			
	Bedtime			

Day	Meal	Before	After	Notes
Wednesday > > >	Breakfast			
	Lunch			
	Dinner			
	Bedtime			

Day	Meal	Before	After	Notes
Thursday > > >	Breakfast			
	Lunch			
	Dinner			
	Bedtime			

Day	Meal	Before	After	Notes
Friday > > >	Breakfast			
	Lunch			
	Dinner			
	Bedtime			

Day	Meal	Before	After	Notes
Saturday > > >	Breakfast			
	Lunch			
	Dinner			
	Bedtime			

Day	Meal	Before	After	Notes
Sunday > > >	Breakfast			
	Lunch			
	Dinner			
	Bedtime			

Weekly Blood Sugar Log

Week: _____   Weight: _____

Day	Meal	Before	After	Notes
Monday > > >	Breakfast			
	Lunch			
	Dinner			
	Bedtime			

Day	Meal	Before	After	Notes
Tuesday > > >	Breakfast			
	Lunch			
	Dinner			
	Bedtime			

Day	Meal	Before	After	Notes
Wednesday > > >	Breakfast			
	Lunch			
	Dinner			
	Bedtime			

Day	Meal	Before	After	Notes
Thursday > > >	Breakfast			
	Lunch			
	Dinner			
	Bedtime			

Day	Meal	Before	After	Notes
Friday > > >	Breakfast			
	Lunch			
	Dinner			
	Bedtime			

Day	Meal	Before	After	Notes
Saturday > > >	Breakfast			
	Lunch			
	Dinner			
	Bedtime			

Day	Meal	Before	After	Notes
Sunday > > >	Breakfast			
	Lunch			
	Dinner			
	Bedtime			

Weekly Blood Sugar Log

Week: _____   Weight: _____

Day	Meal	Before	After	Notes
Monday > > >	Breakfast			
	Lunch			
	Dinner			
	Bedtime			

Day	Meal	Before	After	Notes
Tuesday > > >	Breakfast			
	Lunch			
	Dinner			
	Bedtime			

Day	Meal	Before	After	Notes
Wednesday > > >	Breakfast			
	Lunch			
	Dinner			
	Bedtime			

Day	Meal	Before	After	Notes
Thursday > > >	Breakfast			
	Lunch			
	Dinner			
	Bedtime			

Day	Meal	Before	After	Notes
Friday > > >	Breakfast			
	Lunch			
	Dinner			
	Bedtime			

Day	Meal	Before	After	Notes
Saturday > > >	Breakfast			
	Lunch			
	Dinner			
	Bedtime			

Day	Meal	Before	After	Notes
Sunday > > >	Breakfast			
	Lunch			
	Dinner			
	Bedtime			

Weekly Blood Sugar Log

Week: _____   Weight: _____

Day	Meal	Before	After	Notes
Monday > > >	Breakfast			
	Lunch			
	Dinner			
	Bedtime			

Day	Meal	Before	After	Notes
Tuesday > > >	Breakfast			
	Lunch			
	Dinner			
	Bedtime			

Day	Meal	Before	After	Notes
Wednesday > > >	Breakfast			
	Lunch			
	Dinner			
	Bedtime			

Day	Meal	Before	After	Notes
Thursday > > >	Breakfast			
	Lunch			
	Dinner			
	Bedtime			

Day	Meal	Before	After	Notes
Friday > > >	Breakfast			
	Lunch			
	Dinner			
	Bedtime			

Day	Meal	Before	After	Notes
Saturday > > >	Breakfast			
	Lunch			
	Dinner			
	Bedtime			

Day	Meal	Before	After	Notes
Sunday > > >	Breakfast			
	Lunch			
	Dinner			
	Bedtime			

Weekly Blood Sugar Log

Week: _____   Weight: _____

Day	Meal	Before	After	Notes
Monday > > >	Breakfast			
	Lunch			
	Dinner			
	Bedtime			

Day	Meal	Before	After	Notes
Tuesday > > >	Breakfast			
	Lunch			
	Dinner			
	Bedtime			

Day	Meal	Before	After	Notes
Wednesday > > >	Breakfast			
	Lunch			
	Dinner			
	Bedtime			

Day	Meal	Before	After	Notes
Thursday > > >	Breakfast			
	Lunch			
	Dinner			
	Bedtime			

Day	Meal	Before	After	Notes
Friday > > >	Breakfast			
	Lunch			
	Dinner			
	Bedtime			

Day	Meal	Before	After	Notes
Saturday > > >	Breakfast			
	Lunch			
	Dinner			
	Bedtime			

Day	Meal	Before	After	Notes
Sunday > > >	Breakfast			
	Lunch			
	Dinner			
	Bedtime			

Weekly Blood Sugar Log

Week: _____   Weight: _____

Day	Meal	Before	After	Notes
Monday > > >	Breakfast			
	Lunch			
	Dinner			
	Bedtime			

Day	Meal	Before	After	Notes
Tuesday > > >	Breakfast			
	Lunch			
	Dinner			
	Bedtime			

Day	Meal	Before	After	Notes
Wednesday > > >	Breakfast			
	Lunch			
	Dinner			
	Bedtime			

Day	Meal	Before	After	Notes
Thursday > > >	Breakfast			
	Lunch			
	Dinner			
	Bedtime			

Day	Meal	Before	After	Notes
Friday > > >	Breakfast			
	Lunch			
	Dinner			
	Bedtime			

Day	Meal	Before	After	Notes
Saturday > > >	Breakfast			
	Lunch			
	Dinner			
	Bedtime			

Day	Meal	Before	After	Notes
Sunday > > >	Breakfast			
	Lunch			
	Dinner			
	Bedtime			

Weekly Blood Sugar Log

Week: _____   Weight: _____

Day	Meal	Before	After	Notes
Monday > > >	Breakfast			
	Lunch			
	Dinner			
	Bedtime			

Day	Meal	Before	After	Notes
Tuesday > > >	Breakfast			
	Lunch			
	Dinner			
	Bedtime			

Day	Meal	Before	After	Notes
Wednesday > > >	Breakfast			
	Lunch			
	Dinner			
	Bedtime			

Day	Meal	Before	After	Notes
Thursday > > >	Breakfast			
	Lunch			
	Dinner			
	Bedtime			

Day	Meal	Before	After	Notes
Friday > > >	Breakfast			
	Lunch			
	Dinner			
	Bedtime			

Day	Meal	Before	After	Notes
Saturday > > >	Breakfast			
	Lunch			
	Dinner			
	Bedtime			

Day	Meal	Before	After	Notes
Sunday > > >	Breakfast			
	Lunch			
	Dinner			
	Bedtime			

Weekly Blood Sugar Log

Week: _____   Weight: _____

Day	Meal	Before	After	Notes
Monday > > >	Breakfast			
	Lunch			
	Dinner			
	Bedtime			

Day	Meal	Before	After	Notes
Tuesday > > >	Breakfast			
	Lunch			
	Dinner			
	Bedtime			

Day	Meal	Before	After	Notes
Wednesday > > >	Breakfast			
	Lunch			
	Dinner			
	Bedtime			

Day	Meal	Before	After	Notes
Thursday > > >	Breakfast			
	Lunch			
	Dinner			
	Bedtime			

Day	Meal	Before	After	Notes
Friday > > >	Breakfast			
	Lunch			
	Dinner			
	Bedtime			

Day	Meal	Before	After	Notes
Saturday > > >	Breakfast			
	Lunch			
	Dinner			
	Bedtime			

Day	Meal	Before	After	Notes
Sunday > > >	Breakfast			
	Lunch			
	Dinner			
	Bedtime			

Weekly Blood Sugar Log

Week: _____   Weight: _____

Day	Meal	Before	After	Notes
Monday > > >	Breakfast			
	Lunch			
	Dinner			
	Bedtime			

Day	Meal	Before	After	Notes
Tuesday > > >	Breakfast			
	Lunch			
	Dinner			
	Bedtime			

Day	Meal	Before	After	Notes
Wednesday > > >	Breakfast			
	Lunch			
	Dinner			
	Bedtime			

Day	Meal	Before	After	Notes
Thursday > > >	Breakfast			
	Lunch			
	Dinner			
	Bedtime			

Day	Meal	Before	After	Notes
Friday > > >	Breakfast			
	Lunch			
	Dinner			
	Bedtime			

Day	Meal	Before	After	Notes
Saturday > > >	Breakfast			
	Lunch			
	Dinner			
	Bedtime			

Day	Meal	Before	After	Notes
Sunday > > >	Breakfast			
	Lunch			
	Dinner			
	Bedtime			

Weekly Blood Sugar Log

Week: _____   Weight: _____

Day	Meal	Before	After	Notes
Monday > > >	Breakfast			
	Lunch			
	Dinner			
	Bedtime			

Day	Meal	Before	After	Notes
Tuesday > > >	Breakfast			
	Lunch			
	Dinner			
	Bedtime			

Day	Meal	Before	After	Notes
Wednesday > > >	Breakfast			
	Lunch			
	Dinner			
	Bedtime			

Day	Meal	Before	After	Notes
Thursday > > >	Breakfast			
	Lunch			
	Dinner			
	Bedtime			

Day	Meal	Before	After	Notes
Friday > > >	Breakfast			
	Lunch			
	Dinner			
	Bedtime			

Day	Meal	Before	After	Notes
Saturday > > >	Breakfast			
	Lunch			
	Dinner			
	Bedtime			

Day	Meal	Before	After	Notes
Sunday > > >	Breakfast			
	Lunch			
	Dinner			
	Bedtime			

Weekly Blood Sugar Log

Week: _____   Weight: _____

Day	Meal	Before	After	Notes
Monday > > >	Breakfast			
	Lunch			
	Dinner			
	Bedtime			

Day	Meal	Before	After	Notes
Tuesday > > >	Breakfast			
	Lunch			
	Dinner			
	Bedtime			

Day	Meal	Before	After	Notes
Wednesday > > >	Breakfast			
	Lunch			
	Dinner			
	Bedtime			

Day	Meal	Before	After	Notes
Thursday > > >	Breakfast			
	Lunch			
	Dinner			
	Bedtime			

Day	Meal	Before	After	Notes
Friday > > >	Breakfast			
	Lunch			
	Dinner			
	Bedtime			

Day	Meal	Before	After	Notes
Saturday > > >	Breakfast			
	Lunch			
	Dinner			
	Bedtime			

Day	Meal	Before	After	Notes
Sunday > > >	Breakfast			
	Lunch			
	Dinner			
	Bedtime			

Weekly Blood Sugar Log

Week: _____   Weight: _____

Day	Meal	Before	After	Notes
Monday > > >	Breakfast			
	Lunch			
	Dinner			
	Bedtime			

Day	Meal	Before	After	Notes
Tuesday > > >	Breakfast			
	Lunch			
	Dinner			
	Bedtime			

Day	Meal	Before	After	Notes
Wednesday > > >	Breakfast			
	Lunch			
	Dinner			
	Bedtime			

Day	Meal	Before	After	Notes
Thursday > > >	Breakfast			
	Lunch			
	Dinner			
	Bedtime			

Day	Meal	Before	After	Notes
Friday > > >	Breakfast			
	Lunch			
	Dinner			
	Bedtime			

Day	Meal	Before	After	Notes
Saturday > > >	Breakfast			
	Lunch			
	Dinner			
	Bedtime			

Day	Meal	Before	After	Notes
Sunday > > >	Breakfast			
	Lunch			
	Dinner			
	Bedtime			

Weekly Blood Sugar Log

Week: Weight:

Day	Meal	Before	After	Notes
Monday > > >	Breakfast Lunch Dinner Bedtime			

Day	Meal	Before	After	Notes
Tuesday > > >	Breakfast Lunch Dinner Bedtime			

Day	Meal	Before	After	Notes
Wednesday > > >	Breakfast Lunch Dinner Bedtime			

Day	Meal	Before	After	Notes
Thursday > > >	Breakfast Lunch Dinner Bedtime			

Day	Meal	Before	After	Notes
Friday > > >	Breakfast Lunch Dinner Bedtime			

Day	Meal	Before	After	Notes
Saturday > > >	Breakfast Lunch Dinner Bedtime			

Day	Meal	Before	After	Notes
Sunday > > >	Breakfast Lunch Dinner Bedtime			

Weekly Blood Sugar Log

Week: _____   Weight: _____

Day	Meal	Before	After	Notes
Monday > > >	Breakfast			
	Lunch			
	Dinner			
	Bedtime			

Day	Meal	Before	After	Notes
Tuesday > > >	Breakfast			
	Lunch			
	Dinner			
	Bedtime			

Day	Meal	Before	After	Notes
Wednesday > > >	Breakfast			
	Lunch			
	Dinner			
	Bedtime			

Day	Meal	Before	After	Notes
Thursday > > >	Breakfast			
	Lunch			
	Dinner			
	Bedtime			

Day	Meal	Before	After	Notes
Friday > > >	Breakfast			
	Lunch			
	Dinner			
	Bedtime			

Day	Meal	Before	After	Notes
Saturday > > >	Breakfast			
	Lunch			
	Dinner			
	Bedtime			

Day	Meal	Before	After	Notes
Sunday > > >	Breakfast			
	Lunch			
	Dinner			
	Bedtime			

Weekly Blood Sugar Log

Week: _____   Weight: _____

Day	Meal	Before	After	Notes
Monday > > >	Breakfast			
	Lunch			
	Dinner			
	Bedtime			

Day	Meal	Before	After	Notes
Tuesday > > >	Breakfast			
	Lunch			
	Dinner			
	Bedtime			

Day	Meal	Before	After	Notes
Wednesday > > >	Breakfast			
	Lunch			
	Dinner			
	Bedtime			

Day	Meal	Before	After	Notes
Thursday > > >	Breakfast			
	Lunch			
	Dinner			
	Bedtime			

Day	Meal	Before	After	Notes
Friday > > >	Breakfast			
	Lunch			
	Dinner			
	Bedtime			

Day	Meal	Before	After	Notes
Saturday > > >	Breakfast			
	Lunch			
	Dinner			
	Bedtime			

Day	Meal	Before	After	Notes
Sunday > > >	Breakfast			
	Lunch			
	Dinner			
	Bedtime			

Weekly Blood Sugar Log

Week: _____   Weight: _____

Day	Meal	Before	After	Notes
Monday > > >	Breakfast			
	Lunch			
	Dinner			
	Bedtime			

Day	Meal	Before	After	Notes
Tuesday > > >	Breakfast			
	Lunch			
	Dinner			
	Bedtime			

Day	Meal	Before	After	Notes
Wednesday > > >	Breakfast			
	Lunch			
	Dinner			
	Bedtime			

Day	Meal	Before	After	Notes
Thursday > > >	Breakfast			
	Lunch			
	Dinner			
	Bedtime			

Day	Meal	Before	After	Notes
Friday > > >	Breakfast			
	Lunch			
	Dinner			
	Bedtime			

Day	Meal	Before	After	Notes
Saturday > > >	Breakfast			
	Lunch			
	Dinner			
	Bedtime			

Day	Meal	Before	After	Notes
Sunday > > >	Breakfast			
	Lunch			
	Dinner			
	Bedtime			

Weekly Blood Sugar Log

Week: _____   Weight: _____

Day	Meal	Before	After	Notes
Monday > > >	Breakfast			
	Lunch			
	Dinner			
	Bedtime			

Day	Meal	Before	After	Notes
Tuesday > > >	Breakfast			
	Lunch			
	Dinner			
	Bedtime			

Day	Meal	Before	After	Notes
Wednesday > > >	Breakfast			
	Lunch			
	Dinner			
	Bedtime			

Day	Meal	Before	After	Notes
Thursday > > >	Breakfast			
	Lunch			
	Dinner			
	Bedtime			

Day	Meal	Before	After	Notes
Friday > > >	Breakfast			
	Lunch			
	Dinner			
	Bedtime			

Day	Meal	Before	After	Notes
Saturday > > >	Breakfast			
	Lunch			
	Dinner			
	Bedtime			

Day	Meal	Before	After	Notes
Sunday > > >	Breakfast			
	Lunch			
	Dinner			
	Bedtime			

Weekly Blood Sugar Log

Week: _____   Weight: _____

Day	Meal	Before	After	Notes
Monday > > >	Breakfast			
	Lunch			
	Dinner			
	Bedtime			

Day	Meal	Before	After	Notes
Tuesday > > >	Breakfast			
	Lunch			
	Dinner			
	Bedtime			

Day	Meal	Before	After	Notes
Wednesday > > >	Breakfast			
	Lunch			
	Dinner			
	Bedtime			

Day	Meal	Before	After	Notes
Thursday > > >	Breakfast			
	Lunch			
	Dinner			
	Bedtime			

Day	Meal	Before	After	Notes
Friday > > >	Breakfast			
	Lunch			
	Dinner			
	Bedtime			

Day	Meal	Before	After	Notes
Saturday > > >	Breakfast			
	Lunch			
	Dinner			
	Bedtime			

Day	Meal	Before	After	Notes
Sunday > > >	Breakfast			
	Lunch			
	Dinner			
	Bedtime			

Weekly Blood Sugar Log

Week: Weight:

Day	Meal	Before	After	Notes
Monday > > >	Breakfast			
	Lunch			
	Dinner			
	Bedtime			

Day	Meal	Before	After	Notes
Tuesday > > >	Breakfast			
	Lunch			
	Dinner			
	Bedtime			

Day	Meal	Before	After	Notes
Wednesday > > >	Breakfast			
	Lunch			
	Dinner			
	Bedtime			

Day	Meal	Before	After	Notes
Thursday > > >	Breakfast			
	Lunch			
	Dinner			
	Bedtime			

Day	Meal	Before	After	Notes
Friday > > >	Breakfast			
	Lunch			
	Dinner			
	Bedtime			

Day	Meal	Before	After	Notes
Saturday > > >	Breakfast			
	Lunch			
	Dinner			
	Bedtime			

Day	Meal	Before	After	Notes
Sunday > > >	Breakfast			
	Lunch			
	Dinner			
	Bedtime			

Weekly Blood Sugar Log

Week: _____   Weight: _____

Day	Meal	Before	After	Notes
Monday ＞ ＞ ＞	Breakfast			
	Lunch			
	Dinner			
	Bedtime			

Day	Meal	Before	After	Notes
Tuesday ＞ ＞ ＞	Breakfast			
	Lunch			
	Dinner			
	Bedtime			

Day	Meal	Before	After	Notes
Wednesday ＞ ＞ ＞	Breakfast			
	Lunch			
	Dinner			
	Bedtime			

Day	Meal	Before	After	Notes
Thursday ＞ ＞ ＞	Breakfast			
	Lunch			
	Dinner			
	Bedtime			

Day	Meal	Before	After	Notes
Friday ＞ ＞ ＞	Breakfast			
	Lunch			
	Dinner			
	Bedtime			

Day	Meal	Before	After	Notes
Saturday ＞ ＞ ＞	Breakfast			
	Lunch			
	Dinner			
	Bedtime			

Day	Meal	Before	After	Notes
Sunday ＞ ＞ ＞	Breakfast			
	Lunch			
	Dinner			
	Bedtime			

Weekly Blood Sugar Log

Week: _____   Weight: _____

Day	Meal	Before	After	Notes
Monday > > >	Breakfast			
	Lunch			
	Dinner			
	Bedtime			

Day	Meal	Before	After	Notes
Tuesday > > >	Breakfast			
	Lunch			
	Dinner			
	Bedtime			

Day	Meal	Before	After	Notes
Wednesday > > >	Breakfast			
	Lunch			
	Dinner			
	Bedtime			

Day	Meal	Before	After	Notes
Thursday > > >	Breakfast			
	Lunch			
	Dinner			
	Bedtime			

Day	Meal	Before	After	Notes
Friday > > >	Breakfast			
	Lunch			
	Dinner			
	Bedtime			

Day	Meal	Before	After	Notes
Saturday > > >	Breakfast			
	Lunch			
	Dinner			
	Bedtime			

Day	Meal	Before	After	Notes
Sunday > > >	Breakfast			
	Lunch			
	Dinner			
	Bedtime			

Weekly Blood Sugar Log

Week: _____   Weight: _____

Day	Meal	Before	After	Notes
Monday > > >	Breakfast			
	Lunch			
	Dinner			
	Bedtime			

Day	Meal	Before	After	Notes
Tuesday > > >	Breakfast			
	Lunch			
	Dinner			
	Bedtime			

Day	Meal	Before	After	Notes
Wednesday > > >	Breakfast			
	Lunch			
	Dinner			
	Bedtime			

Day	Meal	Before	After	Notes
Thursday > > >	Breakfast			
	Lunch			
	Dinner			
	Bedtime			

Day	Meal	Before	After	Notes
Friday > > >	Breakfast			
	Lunch			
	Dinner			
	Bedtime			

Day	Meal	Before	After	Notes
Saturday > > >	Breakfast			
	Lunch			
	Dinner			
	Bedtime			

Day	Meal	Before	After	Notes
Sunday > > >	Breakfast			
	Lunch			
	Dinner			
	Bedtime			

Weekly Blood Sugar Log

Week: _____   Weight: _____

Day	Meal	Before	After	Notes
Monday > > >	Breakfast			
	Lunch			
	Dinner			
	Bedtime			

Day	Meal	Before	After	Notes
Tuesday > > >	Breakfast			
	Lunch			
	Dinner			
	Bedtime			

Day	Meal	Before	After	Notes
Wednesday > > >	Breakfast			
	Lunch			
	Dinner			
	Bedtime			

Day	Meal	Before	After	Notes
Thursday > > >	Breakfast			
	Lunch			
	Dinner			
	Bedtime			

Day	Meal	Before	After	Notes
Friday > > >	Breakfast			
	Lunch			
	Dinner			
	Bedtime			

Day	Meal	Before	After	Notes
Saturday > > >	Breakfast			
	Lunch			
	Dinner			
	Bedtime			

Day	Meal	Before	After	Notes
Sunday > > >	Breakfast			
	Lunch			
	Dinner			
	Bedtime			

Weekly Blood Sugar Log

Week: _____   Weight: _____

Day	Meal	Before	After	Notes
Monday > > >	Breakfast			
	Lunch			
	Dinner			
	Bedtime			

Day	Meal	Before	After	Notes
Tuesday > > >	Breakfast			
	Lunch			
	Dinner			
	Bedtime			

Day	Meal	Before	After	Notes
Wednesday > > >	Breakfast			
	Lunch			
	Dinner			
	Bedtime			

Day	Meal	Before	After	Notes
Thursday > > >	Breakfast			
	Lunch			
	Dinner			
	Bedtime			

Day	Meal	Before	After	Notes
Friday > > >	Breakfast			
	Lunch			
	Dinner			
	Bedtime			

Day	Meal	Before	After	Notes
Saturday > > >	Breakfast			
	Lunch			
	Dinner			
	Bedtime			

Day	Meal	Before	After	Notes
Sunday > > >	Breakfast			
	Lunch			
	Dinner			
	Bedtime			

Weekly Blood Sugar Log

Week: _____   Weight: _____

Day	Meal	Before	After	Notes
Monday > > >	Breakfast			
	Lunch			
	Dinner			
	Bedtime			

Day	Meal	Before	After	Notes
Tuesday > > >	Breakfast			
	Lunch			
	Dinner			
	Bedtime			

Day	Meal	Before	After	Notes
Wednesday > > >	Breakfast			
	Lunch			
	Dinner			
	Bedtime			

Day	Meal	Before	After	Notes
Thursday > > >	Breakfast			
	Lunch			
	Dinner			
	Bedtime			

Day	Meal	Before	After	Notes
Friday > > >	Breakfast			
	Lunch			
	Dinner			
	Bedtime			

Day	Meal	Before	After	Notes
Saturday > > >	Breakfast			
	Lunch			
	Dinner			
	Bedtime			

Day	Meal	Before	After	Notes
Sunday > > >	Breakfast			
	Lunch			
	Dinner			
	Bedtime			

Weekly Blood Sugar Log

Week: _____   Weight: _____

Day	Meal	Before	After	Notes
Monday > > >	Breakfast			
	Lunch			
	Dinner			
	Bedtime			

Day	Meal	Before	After	Notes
Tuesday > > >	Breakfast			
	Lunch			
	Dinner			
	Bedtime			

Day	Meal	Before	After	Notes
Wednesday > > >	Breakfast			
	Lunch			
	Dinner			
	Bedtime			

Day	Meal	Before	After	Notes
Thursday > > >	Breakfast			
	Lunch			
	Dinner			
	Bedtime			

Day	Meal	Before	After	Notes
Friday > > >	Breakfast			
	Lunch			
	Dinner			
	Bedtime			

Day	Meal	Before	After	Notes
Saturday > > >	Breakfast			
	Lunch			
	Dinner			
	Bedtime			

Day	Meal	Before	After	Notes
Sunday > > >	Breakfast			
	Lunch			
	Dinner			
	Bedtime			

Weekly Blood Sugar Log

Week: _____   Weight: _____

Day	Meal	Before	After	Notes
Monday	Breakfast			
> > >	Lunch			
	Dinner			
	Bedtime			

Day	Meal	Before	After	Notes
Tuesday	Breakfast			
> > >	Lunch			
	Dinner			
	Bedtime			

Day	Meal	Before	After	Notes
Wednesday	Breakfast			
> > >	Lunch			
	Dinner			
	Bedtime			

Day	Meal	Before	After	Notes
Thursday	Breakfast			
> > >	Lunch			
	Dinner			
	Bedtime			

Day	Meal	Before	After	Notes
Friday	Breakfast			
> > >	Lunch			
	Dinner			
	Bedtime			

Day	Meal	Before	After	Notes
Saturday	Breakfast			
> > >	Lunch			
	Dinner			
	Bedtime			

Day	Meal	Before	After	Notes
Sunday	Breakfast			
> > >	Lunch			
	Dinner			
	Bedtime			

Weekly Blood Sugar Log

Week: _____   Weight: _____

Day	Meal	Before	After	Notes
Monday > > >	Breakfast			
	Lunch			
	Dinner			
	Bedtime			

Day	Meal	Before	After	Notes
Tuesday > > >	Breakfast			
	Lunch			
	Dinner			
	Bedtime			

Day	Meal	Before	After	Notes
Wednesday > > >	Breakfast			
	Lunch			
	Dinner			
	Bedtime			

Day	Meal	Before	After	Notes
Thursday > > >	Breakfast			
	Lunch			
	Dinner			
	Bedtime			

Day	Meal	Before	After	Notes
Friday > > >	Breakfast			
	Lunch			
	Dinner			
	Bedtime			

Day	Meal	Before	After	Notes
Saturday > > >	Breakfast			
	Lunch			
	Dinner			
	Bedtime			

Day	Meal	Before	After	Notes
Sunday > > >	Breakfast			
	Lunch			
	Dinner			
	Bedtime			

Weekly Blood Sugar Log

Week: Weight:

Day	Meal	Before	After	Notes
Monday > > >	Breakfast			
	Lunch			
	Dinner			
	Bedtime			

Day	Meal	Before	After	Notes
Tuesday > > >	Breakfast			
	Lunch			
	Dinner			
	Bedtime			

Day	Meal	Before	After	Notes
Wednesday > > >	Breakfast			
	Lunch			
	Dinner			
	Bedtime			

Day	Meal	Before	After	Notes
Thursday > > >	Breakfast			
	Lunch			
	Dinner			
	Bedtime			

Day	Meal	Before	After	Notes
Friday > > >	Breakfast			
	Lunch			
	Dinner			
	Bedtime			

Day	Meal	Before	After	Notes
Saturday > > >	Breakfast			
	Lunch			
	Dinner			
	Bedtime			

Day	Meal	Before	After	Notes
Sunday > > >	Breakfast			
	Lunch			
	Dinner			
	Bedtime			

Weekly Blood Sugar Log

Week: _____   Weight: _____

Day	Meal	Before	After	Notes
Monday > > >	Breakfast			
	Lunch			
	Dinner			
	Bedtime			

Day	Meal	Before	After	Notes
Tuesday > > >	Breakfast			
	Lunch			
	Dinner			
	Bedtime			

Day	Meal	Before	After	Notes
Wednesday > > >	Breakfast			
	Lunch			
	Dinner			
	Bedtime			

Day	Meal	Before	After	Notes
Thursday > > >	Breakfast			
	Lunch			
	Dinner			
	Bedtime			

Day	Meal	Before	After	Notes
Friday > > >	Breakfast			
	Lunch			
	Dinner			
	Bedtime			

Day	Meal	Before	After	Notes
Saturday > > >	Breakfast			
	Lunch			
	Dinner			
	Bedtime			

Day	Meal	Before	After	Notes
Sunday > > >	Breakfast			
	Lunch			
	Dinner			
	Bedtime			

Weekly Blood Sugar Log

Week: _____   Weight: _____

Day	Meal	Before	After	Notes
Monday > > >	Breakfast			
	Lunch			
	Dinner			
	Bedtime			

Day	Meal	Before	After	Notes
Tuesday > > >	Breakfast			
	Lunch			
	Dinner			
	Bedtime			

Day	Meal	Before	After	Notes
Wednesday > > >	Breakfast			
	Lunch			
	Dinner			
	Bedtime			

Day	Meal	Before	After	Notes
Thursday > > >	Breakfast			
	Lunch			
	Dinner			
	Bedtime			

Day	Meal	Before	After	Notes
Friday > > >	Breakfast			
	Lunch			
	Dinner			
	Bedtime			

Day	Meal	Before	After	Notes
Saturday > > >	Breakfast			
	Lunch			
	Dinner			
	Bedtime			

Day	Meal	Before	After	Notes
Sunday > > >	Breakfast			
	Lunch			
	Dinner			
	Bedtime			

Weekly Blood Sugar Log

Week: _____   Weight: _____

Day	Meal	Before	After	Notes
Monday > > >	Breakfast			
	Lunch			
	Dinner			
	Bedtime			

Day	Meal	Before	After	Notes
Tuesday > > >	Breakfast			
	Lunch			
	Dinner			
	Bedtime			

Day	Meal	Before	After	Notes
Wednesday > > >	Breakfast			
	Lunch			
	Dinner			
	Bedtime			

Day	Meal	Before	After	Notes
Thursday > > >	Breakfast			
	Lunch			
	Dinner			
	Bedtime			

Day	Meal	Before	After	Notes
Friday > > >	Breakfast			
	Lunch			
	Dinner			
	Bedtime			

Day	Meal	Before	After	Notes
Saturday > > >	Breakfast			
	Lunch			
	Dinner			
	Bedtime			

Day	Meal	Before	After	Notes
Sunday > > >	Breakfast			
	Lunch			
	Dinner			
	Bedtime			

Weekly Blood Sugar Log

Week: _____   Weight: _____

Day	Meal	Before	After	Notes
Monday > > >	Breakfast			
	Lunch			
	Dinner			
	Bedtime			

Day	Meal	Before	After	Notes
Tuesday > > >	Breakfast			
	Lunch			
	Dinner			
	Bedtime			

Day	Meal	Before	After	Notes
Wednesday > > >	Breakfast			
	Lunch			
	Dinner			
	Bedtime			

Day	Meal	Before	After	Notes
Thursday > > >	Breakfast			
	Lunch			
	Dinner			
	Bedtime			

Day	Meal	Before	After	Notes
Friday > > >	Breakfast			
	Lunch			
	Dinner			
	Bedtime			

Day	Meal	Before	After	Notes
Saturday > > >	Breakfast			
	Lunch			
	Dinner			
	Bedtime			

Day	Meal	Before	After	Notes
Sunday > > >	Breakfast			
	Lunch			
	Dinner			
	Bedtime			

Weekly Blood Sugar Log

Week: _____ Weight: _____

Day	Meal	Before	After	Notes
Monday > > >	Breakfast			
	Lunch			
	Dinner			
	Bedtime			

Day	Meal	Before	After	Notes
Tuesday > > >	Breakfast			
	Lunch			
	Dinner			
	Bedtime			

Day	Meal	Before	After	Notes
Wednesday > > >	Breakfast			
	Lunch			
	Dinner			
	Bedtime			

Day	Meal	Before	After	Notes
Thursday > > >	Breakfast			
	Lunch			
	Dinner			
	Bedtime			

Day	Meal	Before	After	Notes
Friday > > >	Breakfast			
	Lunch			
	Dinner			
	Bedtime			

Day	Meal	Before	After	Notes
Saturday > > >	Breakfast			
	Lunch			
	Dinner			
	Bedtime			

Day	Meal	Before	After	Notes
Sunday > > >	Breakfast			
	Lunch			
	Dinner			
	Bedtime			

Weekly Blood Sugar Log

Week: _____   Weight: _____

Day	Meal	Before	After	Notes
Monday > > >	Breakfast			
	Lunch			
	Dinner			
	Bedtime			

Day	Meal	Before	After	Notes
Tuesday > > >	Breakfast			
	Lunch			
	Dinner			
	Bedtime			

Day	Meal	Before	After	Notes
Wednesday > > >	Breakfast			
	Lunch			
	Dinner			
	Bedtime			

Day	Meal	Before	After	Notes
Thursday > > >	Breakfast			
	Lunch			
	Dinner			
	Bedtime			

Day	Meal	Before	After	Notes
Friday > > >	Breakfast			
	Lunch			
	Dinner			
	Bedtime			

Day	Meal	Before	After	Notes
Saturday > > >	Breakfast			
	Lunch			
	Dinner			
	Bedtime			

Day	Meal	Before	After	Notes
Sunday > > >	Breakfast			
	Lunch			
	Dinner			
	Bedtime			

Weekly Blood Sugar Log

Week: _____   Weight: _____

Day	Meal	Before	After	Notes
Monday > > >	Breakfast			
	Lunch			
	Dinner			
	Bedtime			

Day	Meal	Before	After	Notes
Tuesday > > >	Breakfast			
	Lunch			
	Dinner			
	Bedtime			

Day	Meal	Before	After	Notes
Wednesday > > >	Breakfast			
	Lunch			
	Dinner			
	Bedtime			

Day	Meal	Before	After	Notes
Thursday > > >	Breakfast			
	Lunch			
	Dinner			
	Bedtime			

Day	Meal	Before	After	Notes
Friday > > >	Breakfast			
	Lunch			
	Dinner			
	Bedtime			

Day	Meal	Before	After	Notes
Saturday > > >	Breakfast			
	Lunch			
	Dinner			
	Bedtime			

Day	Meal	Before	After	Notes
Sunday > > >	Breakfast			
	Lunch			
	Dinner			
	Bedtime			

Weekly Blood Sugar Log

Week: _____   Weight: _____

Day	Meal	Before	After	Notes
Monday > > >	Breakfast			
	Lunch			
	Dinner			
	Bedtime			

Day	Meal	Before	After	Notes
Tuesday > > >	Breakfast			
	Lunch			
	Dinner			
	Bedtime			

Day	Meal	Before	After	Notes
Wednesday > > >	Breakfast			
	Lunch			
	Dinner			
	Bedtime			

Day	Meal	Before	After	Notes
Thursday > > >	Breakfast			
	Lunch			
	Dinner			
	Bedtime			

Day	Meal	Before	After	Notes
Friday > > >	Breakfast			
	Lunch			
	Dinner			
	Bedtime			

Day	Meal	Before	After	Notes
Saturday > > >	Breakfast			
	Lunch			
	Dinner			
	Bedtime			

Day	Meal	Before	After	Notes
Sunday > > >	Breakfast			
	Lunch			
	Dinner			
	Bedtime			

Weekly Blood Sugar Log

Week: _____   Weight: _____

Day	Meal	Before	After	Notes
Monday > > >	Breakfast Lunch Dinner Bedtime			

Day	Meal	Before	After	Notes
Tuesday > > >	Breakfast Lunch Dinner Bedtime			

Day	Meal	Before	After	Notes
Wednesday > > >	Breakfast Lunch Dinner Bedtime			

Day	Meal	Before	After	Notes
Thursday > > >	Breakfast Lunch Dinner Bedtime			

Day	Meal	Before	After	Notes
Friday > > >	Breakfast Lunch Dinner Bedtime			

Day	Meal	Before	After	Notes
Saturday > > >	Breakfast Lunch Dinner Bedtime			

Day	Meal	Before	After	Notes
Sunday > > >	Breakfast Lunch Dinner Bedtime			

Weekly Blood Sugar Log

Week: _____   Weight: _____

Day	Meal	Before	After	Notes
Monday > > >	Breakfast			
	Lunch			
	Dinner			
	Bedtime			

Day	Meal	Before	After	Notes
Tuesday > > >	Breakfast			
	Lunch			
	Dinner			
	Bedtime			

Day	Meal	Before	After	Notes
Wednesday > > >	Breakfast			
	Lunch			
	Dinner			
	Bedtime			

Day	Meal	Before	After	Notes
Thursday > > >	Breakfast			
	Lunch			
	Dinner			
	Bedtime			

Day	Meal	Before	After	Notes
Friday > > >	Breakfast			
	Lunch			
	Dinner			
	Bedtime			

Day	Meal	Before	After	Notes
Saturday > > >	Breakfast			
	Lunch			
	Dinner			
	Bedtime			

Day	Meal	Before	After	Notes
Sunday > > >	Breakfast			
	Lunch			
	Dinner			
	Bedtime			

Weekly Blood Sugar Log

Week: _____   Weight: _____

Day	Meal	Before	After	Notes
Monday > > >	Breakfast			
	Lunch			
	Dinner			
	Bedtime			

Day	Meal	Before	After	Notes
Tuesday > > >	Breakfast			
	Lunch			
	Dinner			
	Bedtime			

Day	Meal	Before	After	Notes
Wednesday > > >	Breakfast			
	Lunch			
	Dinner			
	Bedtime			

Day	Meal	Before	After	Notes
Thursday > > >	Breakfast			
	Lunch			
	Dinner			
	Bedtime			

Day	Meal	Before	After	Notes
Friday > > >	Breakfast			
	Lunch			
	Dinner			
	Bedtime			

Day	Meal	Before	After	Notes
Saturday > > >	Breakfast			
	Lunch			
	Dinner			
	Bedtime			

Day	Meal	Before	After	Notes
Sunday > > >	Breakfast			
	Lunch			
	Dinner			
	Bedtime			

Weekly Blood Sugar Log

Week: _____   Weight: _____

Day	Meal	Before	After	Notes
Monday > > >	Breakfast			
	Lunch			
	Dinner			
	Bedtime			

Day	Meal	Before	After	Notes
Tuesday > > >	Breakfast			
	Lunch			
	Dinner			
	Bedtime			

Day	Meal	Before	After	Notes
Wednesday > > >	Breakfast			
	Lunch			
	Dinner			
	Bedtime			

Day	Meal	Before	After	Notes
Thursday > > >	Breakfast			
	Lunch			
	Dinner			
	Bedtime			

Day	Meal	Before	After	Notes
Friday > > >	Breakfast			
	Lunch			
	Dinner			
	Bedtime			

Day	Meal	Before	After	Notes
Saturday > > >	Breakfast			
	Lunch			
	Dinner			
	Bedtime			

Day	Meal	Before	After	Notes
Sunday > > >	Breakfast			
	Lunch			
	Dinner			
	Bedtime			

Weekly Blood Sugar Log

Week: _____   Weight: _____

Day	Meal	Before	After	Notes
Monday > > >	Breakfast			
	Lunch			
	Dinner			
	Bedtime			

Day	Meal	Before	After	Notes
Tuesday > > >	Breakfast			
	Lunch			
	Dinner			
	Bedtime			

Day	Meal	Before	After	Notes
Wednesday > > >	Breakfast			
	Lunch			
	Dinner			
	Bedtime			

Day	Meal	Before	After	Notes
Thursday > > >	Breakfast			
	Lunch			
	Dinner			
	Bedtime			

Day	Meal	Before	After	Notes
Friday > > >	Breakfast			
	Lunch			
	Dinner			
	Bedtime			

Day	Meal	Before	After	Notes
Saturday > > >	Breakfast			
	Lunch			
	Dinner			
	Bedtime			

Day	Meal	Before	After	Notes
Sunday > > >	Breakfast			
	Lunch			
	Dinner			
	Bedtime			

Weekly Blood Sugar Log

Week: _____   Weight: _____

Day	Meal	Before	After	Notes
Monday > > >	Breakfast Lunch Dinner Bedtime			

Day	Meal	Before	After	Notes
Tuesday > > >	Breakfast Lunch Dinner Bedtime			

Day	Meal	Before	After	Notes
Wednesday > > >	Breakfast Lunch Dinner Bedtime			

Day	Meal	Before	After	Notes
Thursday > > >	Breakfast Lunch Dinner Bedtime			

Day	Meal	Before	After	Notes
Friday > > >	Breakfast Lunch Dinner Bedtime			

Day	Meal	Before	After	Notes
Saturday > > >	Breakfast Lunch Dinner Bedtime			

Day	Meal	Before	After	Notes
Sunday > > >	Breakfast Lunch Dinner Bedtime			

Weekly Blood Sugar Log

Week: _____   Weight: _____

Day	Meal	Before	After	Notes
Monday > > >	Breakfast			
	Lunch			
	Dinner			
	Bedtime			

Day	Meal	Before	After	Notes
Tuesday > > >	Breakfast			
	Lunch			
	Dinner			
	Bedtime			

Day	Meal	Before	After	Notes
Wednesday > > >	Breakfast			
	Lunch			
	Dinner			
	Bedtime			

Day	Meal	Before	After	Notes
Thursday > > >	Breakfast			
	Lunch			
	Dinner			
	Bedtime			

Day	Meal	Before	After	Notes
Friday > > >	Breakfast			
	Lunch			
	Dinner			
	Bedtime			

Day	Meal	Before	After	Notes
Saturday > > >	Breakfast			
	Lunch			
	Dinner			
	Bedtime			

Day	Meal	Before	After	Notes
Sunday > > >	Breakfast			
	Lunch			
	Dinner			
	Bedtime			

Weekly Blood Sugar Log

Week: _____   Weight: _____

Day	Meal	Before	After	Notes
Monday > > >	Breakfast			
	Lunch			
	Dinner			
	Bedtime			

Day	Meal	Before	After	Notes
Tuesday > > >	Breakfast			
	Lunch			
	Dinner			
	Bedtime			

Day	Meal	Before	After	Notes
Wednesday > > >	Breakfast			
	Lunch			
	Dinner			
	Bedtime			

Day	Meal	Before	After	Notes
Thursday > > >	Breakfast			
	Lunch			
	Dinner			
	Bedtime			

Day	Meal	Before	After	Notes
Friday > > >	Breakfast			
	Lunch			
	Dinner			
	Bedtime			

Day	Meal	Before	After	Notes
Saturday > > >	Breakfast			
	Lunch			
	Dinner			
	Bedtime			

Day	Meal	Before	After	Notes
Sunday > > >	Breakfast			
	Lunch			
	Dinner			
	Bedtime			

Weekly Blood Sugar Log

Week: _____   Weight: _____

Day	Meal	Before	After	Notes
Monday > > >	Breakfast			
	Lunch			
	Dinner			
	Bedtime			

Day	Meal	Before	After	Notes
Tuesday > > >	Breakfast			
	Lunch			
	Dinner			
	Bedtime			

Day	Meal	Before	After	Notes
Wednesday > > >	Breakfast			
	Lunch			
	Dinner			
	Bedtime			

Day	Meal	Before	After	Notes
Thursday > > >	Breakfast			
	Lunch			
	Dinner			
	Bedtime			

Day	Meal	Before	After	Notes
Friday > > >	Breakfast			
	Lunch			
	Dinner			
	Bedtime			

Day	Meal	Before	After	Notes
Saturday > > >	Breakfast			
	Lunch			
	Dinner			
	Bedtime			

Day	Meal	Before	After	Notes
Sunday > > >	Breakfast			
	Lunch			
	Dinner			
	Bedtime			

Weekly Blood Sugar Log

Week: _____   Weight: _____

Day	Meal	Before	After	Notes
Monday > > >	Breakfast			
	Lunch			
	Dinner			
	Bedtime			

Day	Meal	Before	After	Notes
Tuesday > > >	Breakfast			
	Lunch			
	Dinner			
	Bedtime			

Day	Meal	Before	After	Notes
Wednesday > > >	Breakfast			
	Lunch			
	Dinner			
	Bedtime			

Day	Meal	Before	After	Notes
Thursday > > >	Breakfast			
	Lunch			
	Dinner			
	Bedtime			

Day	Meal	Before	After	Notes
Friday > > >	Breakfast			
	Lunch			
	Dinner			
	Bedtime			

Day	Meal	Before	After	Notes
Saturday > > >	Breakfast			
	Lunch			
	Dinner			
	Bedtime			

Day	Meal	Before	After	Notes
Sunday > > >	Breakfast			
	Lunch			
	Dinner			
	Bedtime			

Weekly Blood Sugar Log

Week: _____ Weight: _____

Day	Meal	Before	After	Notes
Monday > > >	Breakfast			
	Lunch			
	Dinner			
	Bedtime			

Day	Meal	Before	After	Notes
Tuesday > > >	Breakfast			
	Lunch			
	Dinner			
	Bedtime			

Day	Meal	Before	After	Notes
Wednesday > > >	Breakfast			
	Lunch			
	Dinner			
	Bedtime			

Day	Meal	Before	After	Notes
Thursday > > >	Breakfast			
	Lunch			
	Dinner			
	Bedtime			

Day	Meal	Before	After	Notes
Friday > > >	Breakfast			
	Lunch			
	Dinner			
	Bedtime			

Day	Meal	Before	After	Notes
Saturday > > >	Breakfast			
	Lunch			
	Dinner			
	Bedtime			

Day	Meal	Before	After	Notes
Sunday > > >	Breakfast			
	Lunch			
	Dinner			
	Bedtime			

Weekly Blood Sugar Log

Week: _____   Weight: _____

Day	Meal	Before	After	Notes
Monday > > >	Breakfast			
	Lunch			
	Dinner			
	Bedtime			

Day	Meal	Before	After	Notes
Tuesday > > >	Breakfast			
	Lunch			
	Dinner			
	Bedtime			

Day	Meal	Before	After	Notes
Wednesday > > >	Breakfast			
	Lunch			
	Dinner			
	Bedtime			

Day	Meal	Before	After	Notes
Thursday > > >	Breakfast			
	Lunch			
	Dinner			
	Bedtime			

Day	Meal	Before	After	Notes
Friday > > >	Breakfast			
	Lunch			
	Dinner			
	Bedtime			

Day	Meal	Before	After	Notes
Saturday > > >	Breakfast			
	Lunch			
	Dinner			
	Bedtime			

Day	Meal	Before	After	Notes
Sunday > > >	Breakfast			
	Lunch			
	Dinner			
	Bedtime			

Weekly Blood Sugar Log

Week: _____   Weight: _____

Day	Meal	Before	After	Notes
Monday > > >	Breakfast Lunch Dinner Bedtime			

Day	Meal	Before	After	Notes
Tuesday > > >	Breakfast Lunch Dinner Bedtime			

Day	Meal	Before	After	Notes
Wednesday > > >	Breakfast Lunch Dinner Bedtime			

Day	Meal	Before	After	Notes
Thursday > > >	Breakfast Lunch Dinner Bedtime			

Day	Meal	Before	After	Notes
Friday > > >	Breakfast Lunch Dinner Bedtime			

Day	Meal	Before	After	Notes
Saturday > > >	Breakfast Lunch Dinner Bedtime			

Day	Meal	Before	After	Notes
Sunday > > >	Breakfast Lunch Dinner Bedtime			

Weekly Blood Sugar Log

Week: _____   Weight: _____

Day	Meal	Before	After	Notes
Monday > > >	Breakfast			
	Lunch			
	Dinner			
	Bedtime			

Day	Meal	Before	After	Notes
Tuesday > > >	Breakfast			
	Lunch			
	Dinner			
	Bedtime			

Day	Meal	Before	After	Notes
Wednesday > > >	Breakfast			
	Lunch			
	Dinner			
	Bedtime			

Day	Meal	Before	After	Notes
Thursday > > >	Breakfast			
	Lunch			
	Dinner			
	Bedtime			

Day	Meal	Before	After	Notes
Friday > > >	Breakfast			
	Lunch			
	Dinner			
	Bedtime			

Day	Meal	Before	After	Notes
Saturday > > >	Breakfast			
	Lunch			
	Dinner			
	Bedtime			

Day	Meal	Before	After	Notes
Sunday > > >	Breakfast			
	Lunch			
	Dinner			
	Bedtime			

Weekly Blood Sugar Log

Week: _____   Weight: _____

Day	Meal	Before	After	Notes
Monday > > >	Breakfast			
	Lunch			
	Dinner			
	Bedtime			

Day	Meal	Before	After	Notes
Tuesday > > >	Breakfast			
	Lunch			
	Dinner			
	Bedtime			

Day	Meal	Before	After	Notes
Wednesday > > >	Breakfast			
	Lunch			
	Dinner			
	Bedtime			

Day	Meal	Before	After	Notes
Thursday > > >	Breakfast			
	Lunch			
	Dinner			
	Bedtime			

Day	Meal	Before	After	Notes
Friday > > >	Breakfast			
	Lunch			
	Dinner			
	Bedtime			

Day	Meal	Before	After	Notes
Saturday > > >	Breakfast			
	Lunch			
	Dinner			
	Bedtime			

Day	Meal	Before	After	Notes
Sunday > > >	Breakfast			
	Lunch			
	Dinner			
	Bedtime			

Weekly Blood Sugar Log

Week: _____   Weight: _____

Day	Meal	Before	After	Notes
Monday > > >	Breakfast			
	Lunch			
	Dinner			
	Bedtime			

Day	Meal	Before	After	Notes
Tuesday > > >	Breakfast			
	Lunch			
	Dinner			
	Bedtime			

Day	Meal	Before	After	Notes
Wednesday > > >	Breakfast			
	Lunch			
	Dinner			
	Bedtime			

Day	Meal	Before	After	Notes
Thursday > > >	Breakfast			
	Lunch			
	Dinner			
	Bedtime			

Day	Meal	Before	After	Notes
Friday > > >	Breakfast			
	Lunch			
	Dinner			
	Bedtime			

Day	Meal	Before	After	Notes
Saturday > > >	Breakfast			
	Lunch			
	Dinner			
	Bedtime			

Day	Meal	Before	After	Notes
Sunday > > >	Breakfast			
	Lunch			
	Dinner			
	Bedtime			

Weekly Blood Sugar Log

Week: _____   Weight: _____

Day	Meal	Before	After	Notes
Monday > > >	Breakfast			
	Lunch			
	Dinner			
	Bedtime			

Day	Meal	Before	After	Notes
Tuesday > > >	Breakfast			
	Lunch			
	Dinner			
	Bedtime			

Day	Meal	Before	After	Notes
Wednesday > > >	Breakfast			
	Lunch			
	Dinner			
	Bedtime			

Day	Meal	Before	After	Notes
Thursday > > >	Breakfast			
	Lunch			
	Dinner			
	Bedtime			

Day	Meal	Before	After	Notes
Friday > > >	Breakfast			
	Lunch			
	Dinner			
	Bedtime			

Day	Meal	Before	After	Notes
Saturday > > >	Breakfast			
	Lunch			
	Dinner			
	Bedtime			

Day	Meal	Before	After	Notes
Sunday > > >	Breakfast			
	Lunch			
	Dinner			
	Bedtime			

Weekly Blood Sugar Log

Week: _____   Weight: _____

Day	Meal	Before	After	Notes
Monday > > >	Breakfast			
	Lunch			
	Dinner			
	Bedtime			

Day	Meal	Before	After	Notes
Tuesday > > >	Breakfast			
	Lunch			
	Dinner			
	Bedtime			

Day	Meal	Before	After	Notes
Wednesday > > >	Breakfast			
	Lunch			
	Dinner			
	Bedtime			

Day	Meal	Before	After	Notes
Thursday > > >	Breakfast			
	Lunch			
	Dinner			
	Bedtime			

Day	Meal	Before	After	Notes
Friday > > >	Breakfast			
	Lunch			
	Dinner			
	Bedtime			

Day	Meal	Before	After	Notes
Saturday > > >	Breakfast			
	Lunch			
	Dinner			
	Bedtime			

Day	Meal	Before	After	Notes
Sunday > > >	Breakfast			
	Lunch			
	Dinner			
	Bedtime			

Weekly Blood Sugar Log

Week: _____   Weight: _____

Day	Meal	Before	After	Notes
Monday > > >	Breakfast			
	Lunch			
	Dinner			
	Bedtime			

Day	Meal	Before	After	Notes
Tuesday > > >	Breakfast			
	Lunch			
	Dinner			
	Bedtime			

Day	Meal	Before	After	Notes
Wednesday > > >	Breakfast			
	Lunch			
	Dinner			
	Bedtime			

Day	Meal	Before	After	Notes
Thursday > > >	Breakfast			
	Lunch			
	Dinner			
	Bedtime			

Day	Meal	Before	After	Notes
Friday > > >	Breakfast			
	Lunch			
	Dinner			
	Bedtime			

Day	Meal	Before	After	Notes
Saturday > > >	Breakfast			
	Lunch			
	Dinner			
	Bedtime			

Day	Meal	Before	After	Notes
Sunday > > >	Breakfast			
	Lunch			
	Dinner			
	Bedtime			

Weekly Blood Sugar Log

Week: _____   Weight: _____

Day	Meal	Before	After	Notes
Monday > > >	Breakfast			
	Lunch			
	Dinner			
	Bedtime			

Day	Meal	Before	After	Notes
Tuesday > > >	Breakfast			
	Lunch			
	Dinner			
	Bedtime			

Day	Meal	Before	After	Notes
Wednesday > > >	Breakfast			
	Lunch			
	Dinner			
	Bedtime			

Day	Meal	Before	After	Notes
Thursday > > >	Breakfast			
	Lunch			
	Dinner			
	Bedtime			

Day	Meal	Before	After	Notes
Friday > > >	Breakfast			
	Lunch			
	Dinner			
	Bedtime			

Day	Meal	Before	After	Notes
Saturday > > >	Breakfast			
	Lunch			
	Dinner			
	Bedtime			

Day	Meal	Before	After	Notes
Sunday > > >	Breakfast			
	Lunch			
	Dinner			
	Bedtime			

Weekly Blood Sugar Log

Week: _____   Weight: _____

Day	Meal	Before	After	Notes
Monday > > >	Breakfast			
	Lunch			
	Dinner			
	Bedtime			

Day	Meal	Before	After	Notes
Tuesday > > >	Breakfast			
	Lunch			
	Dinner			
	Bedtime			

Day	Meal	Before	After	Notes
Wednesday > > >	Breakfast			
	Lunch			
	Dinner			
	Bedtime			

Day	Meal	Before	After	Notes
Thursday > > >	Breakfast			
	Lunch			
	Dinner			
	Bedtime			

Day	Meal	Before	After	Notes
Friday > > >	Breakfast			
	Lunch			
	Dinner			
	Bedtime			

Day	Meal	Before	After	Notes
Saturday > > >	Breakfast			
	Lunch			
	Dinner			
	Bedtime			

Day	Meal	Before	After	Notes
Sunday > > >	Breakfast			
	Lunch			
	Dinner			
	Bedtime			

Weekly Blood Sugar Log

Week: _____   Weight: _____

Day	Meal	Before	After	Notes
Monday > > >	Breakfast			
	Lunch			
	Dinner			
	Bedtime			

Day	Meal	Before	After	Notes
Tuesday > > >	Breakfast			
	Lunch			
	Dinner			
	Bedtime			

Day	Meal	Before	After	Notes
Wednesday > > >	Breakfast			
	Lunch			
	Dinner			
	Bedtime			

Day	Meal	Before	After	Notes
Thursday > > >	Breakfast			
	Lunch			
	Dinner			
	Bedtime			

Day	Meal	Before	After	Notes
Friday > > >	Breakfast			
	Lunch			
	Dinner			
	Bedtime			

Day	Meal	Before	After	Notes
Saturday > > >	Breakfast			
	Lunch			
	Dinner			
	Bedtime			

Day	Meal	Before	After	Notes
Sunday > > >	Breakfast			
	Lunch			
	Dinner			
	Bedtime			

Weekly Blood Sugar Log

Week: _____   Weight: _____

Day	Meal	Before	After	Notes
Monday > > >	Breakfast			
	Lunch			
	Dinner			
	Bedtime			

Day	Meal	Before	After	Notes
Tuesday > > >	Breakfast			
	Lunch			
	Dinner			
	Bedtime			

Day	Meal	Before	After	Notes
Wednesday > > >	Breakfast			
	Lunch			
	Dinner			
	Bedtime			

Day	Meal	Before	After	Notes
Thursday > > >	Breakfast			
	Lunch			
	Dinner			
	Bedtime			

Day	Meal	Before	After	Notes
Friday > > >	Breakfast			
	Lunch			
	Dinner			
	Bedtime			

Day	Meal	Before	After	Notes
Saturday > > >	Breakfast			
	Lunch			
	Dinner			
	Bedtime			

Day	Meal	Before	After	Notes
Sunday > > >	Breakfast			
	Lunch			
	Dinner			
	Bedtime			

Weekly Blood Sugar Log

Week: _____   Weight: _____

Day	Meal	Before	After	Notes
Monday > > >	Breakfast			
	Lunch			
	Dinner			
	Bedtime			

Day	Meal	Before	After	Notes
Tuesday > > >	Breakfast			
	Lunch			
	Dinner			
	Bedtime			

Day	Meal	Before	After	Notes
Wednesday > > >	Breakfast			
	Lunch			
	Dinner			
	Bedtime			

Day	Meal	Before	After	Notes
Thursday > > >	Breakfast			
	Lunch			
	Dinner			
	Bedtime			

Day	Meal	Before	After	Notes
Friday > > >	Breakfast			
	Lunch			
	Dinner			
	Bedtime			

Day	Meal	Before	After	Notes
Saturday > > >	Breakfast			
	Lunch			
	Dinner			
	Bedtime			

Day	Meal	Before	After	Notes
Sunday > > >	Breakfast			
	Lunch			
	Dinner			
	Bedtime			

Weekly Blood Sugar Log

Week: _____   Weight: _____

Day	Meal	Before	After	Notes
Monday > > >	Breakfast			
	Lunch			
	Dinner			
	Bedtime			

Day	Meal	Before	After	Notes
Tuesday > > >	Breakfast			
	Lunch			
	Dinner			
	Bedtime			

Day	Meal	Before	After	Notes
Wednesday > > >	Breakfast			
	Lunch			
	Dinner			
	Bedtime			

Day	Meal	Before	After	Notes
Thursday > > >	Breakfast			
	Lunch			
	Dinner			
	Bedtime			

Day	Meal	Before	After	Notes
Friday > > >	Breakfast			
	Lunch			
	Dinner			
	Bedtime			

Day	Meal	Before	After	Notes
Saturday > > >	Breakfast			
	Lunch			
	Dinner			
	Bedtime			

Day	Meal	Before	After	Notes
Sunday > > >	Breakfast			
	Lunch			
	Dinner			
	Bedtime			

Weekly Blood Sugar Log

Week: _____   Weight: _____

Day	Meal	Before	After	Notes
Monday > > >	Breakfast			
	Lunch			
	Dinner			
	Bedtime			

Day	Meal	Before	After	Notes
Tuesday > > >	Breakfast			
	Lunch			
	Dinner			
	Bedtime			

Day	Meal	Before	After	Notes
Wednesday > > >	Breakfast			
	Lunch			
	Dinner			
	Bedtime			

Day	Meal	Before	After	Notes
Thursday > > >	Breakfast			
	Lunch			
	Dinner			
	Bedtime			

Day	Meal	Before	After	Notes
Friday > > >	Breakfast			
	Lunch			
	Dinner			
	Bedtime			

Day	Meal	Before	After	Notes
Saturday > > >	Breakfast			
	Lunch			
	Dinner			
	Bedtime			

Day	Meal	Before	After	Notes
Sunday > > >	Breakfast			
	Lunch			
	Dinner			
	Bedtime			

Weekly Blood Sugar Log

Week: _____   Weight: _____

Day	Meal	Before	After	Notes
Monday > > >	Breakfast			
	Lunch			
	Dinner			
	Bedtime			

Day	Meal	Before	After	Notes
Tuesday > > >	Breakfast			
	Lunch			
	Dinner			
	Bedtime			

Day	Meal	Before	After	Notes
Wednesday > > >	Breakfast			
	Lunch			
	Dinner			
	Bedtime			

Day	Meal	Before	After	Notes
Thursday > > >	Breakfast			
	Lunch			
	Dinner			
	Bedtime			

Day	Meal	Before	After	Notes
Friday > > >	Breakfast			
	Lunch			
	Dinner			
	Bedtime			

Day	Meal	Before	After	Notes
Saturday > > >	Breakfast			
	Lunch			
	Dinner			
	Bedtime			

Day	Meal	Before	After	Notes
Sunday > > >	Breakfast			
	Lunch			
	Dinner			
	Bedtime			

Weekly Blood Sugar Log

Week: _____   Weight: _____

Day	Meal	Before	After	Notes
Monday > > >	Breakfast			
	Lunch			
	Dinner			
	Bedtime			

Day	Meal	Before	After	Notes
Tuesday > > >	Breakfast			
	Lunch			
	Dinner			
	Bedtime			

Day	Meal	Before	After	Notes
Wednesday > > >	Breakfast			
	Lunch			
	Dinner			
	Bedtime			

Day	Meal	Before	After	Notes
Thursday > > >	Breakfast			
	Lunch			
	Dinner			
	Bedtime			

Day	Meal	Before	After	Notes
Friday > > >	Breakfast			
	Lunch			
	Dinner			
	Bedtime			

Day	Meal	Before	After	Notes
Saturday > > >	Breakfast			
	Lunch			
	Dinner			
	Bedtime			

Day	Meal	Before	After	Notes
Sunday > > >	Breakfast			
	Lunch			
	Dinner			
	Bedtime			

Weekly Blood Sugar Log

Week: _____   Weight: _____

Day	Meal	Before	After	Notes
Monday > > >	Breakfast			
	Lunch			
	Dinner			
	Bedtime			

Day	Meal	Before	After	Notes
Tuesday > > >	Breakfast			
	Lunch			
	Dinner			
	Bedtime			

Day	Meal	Before	After	Notes
Wednesday > > >	Breakfast			
	Lunch			
	Dinner			
	Bedtime			

Day	Meal	Before	After	Notes
Thursday > > >	Breakfast			
	Lunch			
	Dinner			
	Bedtime			

Day	Meal	Before	After	Notes
Friday > > >	Breakfast			
	Lunch			
	Dinner			
	Bedtime			

Day	Meal	Before	After	Notes
Saturday > > >	Breakfast			
	Lunch			
	Dinner			
	Bedtime			

Day	Meal	Before	After	Notes
Sunday > > >	Breakfast			
	Lunch			
	Dinner			
	Bedtime			

Weekly Blood Sugar Log

Week: _____   Weight: _____

Day	Meal	Before	After	Notes
Monday > > >	Breakfast			
	Lunch			
	Dinner			
	Bedtime			

Day	Meal	Before	After	Notes
Tuesday > > >	Breakfast			
	Lunch			
	Dinner			
	Bedtime			

Day	Meal	Before	After	Notes
Wednesday > > >	Breakfast			
	Lunch			
	Dinner			
	Bedtime			

Day	Meal	Before	After	Notes
Thursday > > >	Breakfast			
	Lunch			
	Dinner			
	Bedtime			

Day	Meal	Before	After	Notes
Friday > > >	Breakfast			
	Lunch			
	Dinner			
	Bedtime			

Day	Meal	Before	After	Notes
Saturday > > >	Breakfast			
	Lunch			
	Dinner			
	Bedtime			

Day	Meal	Before	After	Notes
Sunday > > >	Breakfast			
	Lunch			
	Dinner			
	Bedtime			

Weekly Blood Sugar Log

Week: _____   Weight: _____

Day	Meal	Before	After	Notes
Monday > > >	Breakfast			
	Lunch			
	Dinner			
	Bedtime			

Day	Meal	Before	After	Notes
Tuesday > > >	Breakfast			
	Lunch			
	Dinner			
	Bedtime			

Day	Meal	Before	After	Notes
Wednesday > > >	Breakfast			
	Lunch			
	Dinner			
	Bedtime			

Day	Meal	Before	After	Notes
Thursday > > >	Breakfast			
	Lunch			
	Dinner			
	Bedtime			

Day	Meal	Before	After	Notes
Friday > > >	Breakfast			
	Lunch			
	Dinner			
	Bedtime			

Day	Meal	Before	After	Notes
Saturday > > >	Breakfast			
	Lunch			
	Dinner			
	Bedtime			

Day	Meal	Before	After	Notes
Sunday > > >	Breakfast			
	Lunch			
	Dinner			
	Bedtime			

Weekly Blood Sugar Log

Week: _____   Weight: _____

Day	Meal	Before	After	Notes
Monday > > >	Breakfast			
	Lunch			
	Dinner			
	Bedtime			

Day	Meal	Before	After	Notes
Tuesday > > >	Breakfast			
	Lunch			
	Dinner			
	Bedtime			

Day	Meal	Before	After	Notes
Wednesday > > >	Breakfast			
	Lunch			
	Dinner			
	Bedtime			

Day	Meal	Before	After	Notes
Thursday > > >	Breakfast			
	Lunch			
	Dinner			
	Bedtime			

Day	Meal	Before	After	Notes
Friday > > >	Breakfast			
	Lunch			
	Dinner			
	Bedtime			

Day	Meal	Before	After	Notes
Saturday > > >	Breakfast			
	Lunch			
	Dinner			
	Bedtime			

Day	Meal	Before	After	Notes
Sunday > > >	Breakfast			
	Lunch			
	Dinner			
	Bedtime			

Weekly Blood Sugar Log

Week: _____   Weight: _____

Day	Meal	Before	After	Notes
Monday > > >	Breakfast			
	Lunch			
	Dinner			
	Bedtime			

Day	Meal	Before	After	Notes
Tuesday > > >	Breakfast			
	Lunch			
	Dinner			
	Bedtime			

Day	Meal	Before	After	Notes
Wednesday > > >	Breakfast			
	Lunch			
	Dinner			
	Bedtime			

Day	Meal	Before	After	Notes
Thursday > > >	Breakfast			
	Lunch			
	Dinner			
	Bedtime			

Day	Meal	Before	After	Notes
Friday > > >	Breakfast			
	Lunch			
	Dinner			
	Bedtime			

Day	Meal	Before	After	Notes
Saturday > > >	Breakfast			
	Lunch			
	Dinner			
	Bedtime			

Day	Meal	Before	After	Notes
Sunday > > >	Breakfast			
	Lunch			
	Dinner			
	Bedtime			

Weekly Blood Sugar Log

Week: Weight:

Day	Meal	Before	After	Notes
Monday > > >	Breakfast			
	Lunch			
	Dinner			
	Bedtime			

Day	Meal	Before	After	Notes
Tuesday > > >	Breakfast			
	Lunch			
	Dinner			
	Bedtime			

Day	Meal	Before	After	Notes
Wednesday > > >	Breakfast			
	Lunch			
	Dinner			
	Bedtime			

Day	Meal	Before	After	Notes
Thursday > > >	Breakfast			
	Lunch			
	Dinner			
	Bedtime			

Day	Meal	Before	After	Notes
Friday > > >	Breakfast			
	Lunch			
	Dinner			
	Bedtime			

Day	Meal	Before	After	Notes
Saturday > > >	Breakfast			
	Lunch			
	Dinner			
	Bedtime			

Day	Meal	Before	After	Notes
Sunday > > >	Breakfast			
	Lunch			
	Dinner			
	Bedtime			

Weekly Blood Sugar Log

Week: _____   Weight: _____

Day	Meal	Before	After	Notes
Monday > > >	Breakfast			
	Lunch			
	Dinner			
	Bedtime			

Day	Meal	Before	After	Notes
Tuesday > > >	Breakfast			
	Lunch			
	Dinner			
	Bedtime			

Day	Meal	Before	After	Notes
Wednesday > > >	Breakfast			
	Lunch			
	Dinner			
	Bedtime			

Day	Meal	Before	After	Notes
Thursday > > >	Breakfast			
	Lunch			
	Dinner			
	Bedtime			

Day	Meal	Before	After	Notes
Friday > > >	Breakfast			
	Lunch			
	Dinner			
	Bedtime			

Day	Meal	Before	After	Notes
Saturday > > >	Breakfast			
	Lunch			
	Dinner			
	Bedtime			

Day	Meal	Before	After	Notes
Sunday > > >	Breakfast			
	Lunch			
	Dinner			
	Bedtime			

Weekly Blood Sugar Log

Week: _____   Weight: _____

Day	Meal	Before	After	Notes
Monday > > >	Breakfast			
	Lunch			
	Dinner			
	Bedtime			

Day	Meal	Before	After	Notes
Tuesday > > >	Breakfast			
	Lunch			
	Dinner			
	Bedtime			

Day	Meal	Before	After	Notes
Wednesday > > >	Breakfast			
	Lunch			
	Dinner			
	Bedtime			

Day	Meal	Before	After	Notes
Thursday > > >	Breakfast			
	Lunch			
	Dinner			
	Bedtime			

Day	Meal	Before	After	Notes
Friday > > >	Breakfast			
	Lunch			
	Dinner			
	Bedtime			

Day	Meal	Before	After	Notes
Saturday > > >	Breakfast			
	Lunch			
	Dinner			
	Bedtime			

Day	Meal	Before	After	Notes
Sunday > > >	Breakfast			
	Lunch			
	Dinner			
	Bedtime			

Weekly Blood Sugar Log

Week: _____   Weight: _____

Day	Meal	Before	After	Notes
Monday > > >	Breakfast			
	Lunch			
	Dinner			
	Bedtime			

Day	Meal	Before	After	Notes
Tuesday > > >	Breakfast			
	Lunch			
	Dinner			
	Bedtime			

Day	Meal	Before	After	Notes
Wednesday > > >	Breakfast			
	Lunch			
	Dinner			
	Bedtime			

Day	Meal	Before	After	Notes
Thursday > > >	Breakfast			
	Lunch			
	Dinner			
	Bedtime			

Day	Meal	Before	After	Notes
Friday > > >	Breakfast			
	Lunch			
	Dinner			
	Bedtime			

Day	Meal	Before	After	Notes
Saturday > > >	Breakfast			
	Lunch			
	Dinner			
	Bedtime			

Day	Meal	Before	After	Notes
Sunday > > >	Breakfast			
	Lunch			
	Dinner			
	Bedtime			

Weekly Blood Sugar Log

Week: _____   Weight: _____

Day	Meal	Before	After	Notes
Monday > > >	Breakfast Lunch Dinner Bedtime			

Day	Meal	Before	After	Notes
Tuesday > > >	Breakfast Lunch Dinner Bedtime			

Day	Meal	Before	After	Notes
Wednesday > > >	Breakfast Lunch Dinner Bedtime			

Day	Meal	Before	After	Notes
Thursday > > >	Breakfast Lunch Dinner Bedtime			

Day	Meal	Before	After	Notes
Friday > > >	Breakfast Lunch Dinner Bedtime			

Day	Meal	Before	After	Notes
Saturday > > >	Breakfast Lunch Dinner Bedtime			

Day	Meal	Before	After	Notes
Sunday > > >	Breakfast Lunch Dinner Bedtime			

Weekly Blood Sugar Log

Week: _____   Weight: _____

Day	Meal	Before	After	Notes
Monday > > >	Breakfast			
	Lunch			
	Dinner			
	Bedtime			

Day	Meal	Before	After	Notes
Tuesday > > >	Breakfast			
	Lunch			
	Dinner			
	Bedtime			

Day	Meal	Before	After	Notes
Wednesday > > >	Breakfast			
	Lunch			
	Dinner			
	Bedtime			

Day	Meal	Before	After	Notes
Thursday > > >	Breakfast			
	Lunch			
	Dinner			
	Bedtime			

Day	Meal	Before	After	Notes
Friday > > >	Breakfast			
	Lunch			
	Dinner			
	Bedtime			

Day	Meal	Before	After	Notes
Saturday > > >	Breakfast			
	Lunch			
	Dinner			
	Bedtime			

Day	Meal	Before	After	Notes
Sunday > > >	Breakfast			
	Lunch			
	Dinner			
	Bedtime			

Weekly Blood Sugar Log

Week: ▨▨▨▨▨▨   Weight: ▨▨▨▨▨▨

Day	Meal	Before	After	Notes
Monday > > >	Breakfast			
	Lunch			
	Dinner			
	Bedtime			

Day	Meal	Before	After	Notes
Tuesday > > >	Breakfast			
	Lunch			
	Dinner			
	Bedtime			

Day	Meal	Before	After	Notes
Wednesday > > >	Breakfast			
	Lunch			
	Dinner			
	Bedtime			

Day	Meal	Before	After	Notes
Thursday > > >	Breakfast			
	Lunch			
	Dinner			
	Bedtime			

Day	Meal	Before	After	Notes
Friday > > >	Breakfast			
	Lunch			
	Dinner			
	Bedtime			

Day	Meal	Before	After	Notes
Saturday > > >	Breakfast			
	Lunch			
	Dinner			
	Bedtime			

Day	Meal	Before	After	Notes
Sunday > > >	Breakfast			
	Lunch			
	Dinner			
	Bedtime			

Weekly Blood Sugar Log

Week: _____   Weight: _____

Day	Meal	Before	After	Notes
Monday > > >	Breakfast			
	Lunch			
	Dinner			
	Bedtime			

Day	Meal	Before	After	Notes
Tuesday > > >	Breakfast			
	Lunch			
	Dinner			
	Bedtime			

Day	Meal	Before	After	Notes
Wednesday > > >	Breakfast			
	Lunch			
	Dinner			
	Bedtime			

Day	Meal	Before	After	Notes
Thursday > > >	Breakfast			
	Lunch			
	Dinner			
	Bedtime			

Day	Meal	Before	After	Notes
Friday > > >	Breakfast			
	Lunch			
	Dinner			
	Bedtime			

Day	Meal	Before	After	Notes
Saturday > > >	Breakfast			
	Lunch			
	Dinner			
	Bedtime			

Day	Meal	Before	After	Notes
Sunday > > >	Breakfast			
	Lunch			
	Dinner			
	Bedtime			

Weekly Blood Sugar Log

Week: _____   Weight: _____

Day	Meal	Before	After	Notes
Monday > > >	Breakfast			
	Lunch			
	Dinner			
	Bedtime			

Day	Meal	Before	After	Notes
Tuesday > > >	Breakfast			
	Lunch			
	Dinner			
	Bedtime			

Day	Meal	Before	After	Notes
Wednesday > > >	Breakfast			
	Lunch			
	Dinner			
	Bedtime			

Day	Meal	Before	After	Notes
Thursday > > >	Breakfast			
	Lunch			
	Dinner			
	Bedtime			

Day	Meal	Before	After	Notes
Friday > > >	Breakfast			
	Lunch			
	Dinner			
	Bedtime			

Day	Meal	Before	After	Notes
Saturday > > >	Breakfast			
	Lunch			
	Dinner			
	Bedtime			

Day	Meal	Before	After	Notes
Sunday > > >	Breakfast			
	Lunch			
	Dinner			
	Bedtime			

Weekly Blood Sugar Log

Week: _____   Weight: _____

Day	Meal	Before	After	Notes
Monday > > >	Breakfast			
	Lunch			
	Dinner			
	Bedtime			

Day	Meal	Before	After	Notes
Tuesday > > >	Breakfast			
	Lunch			
	Dinner			
	Bedtime			

Day	Meal	Before	After	Notes
Wednesday > > >	Breakfast			
	Lunch			
	Dinner			
	Bedtime			

Day	Meal	Before	After	Notes
Thursday > > >	Breakfast			
	Lunch			
	Dinner			
	Bedtime			

Day	Meal	Before	After	Notes
Friday > > >	Breakfast			
	Lunch			
	Dinner			
	Bedtime			

Day	Meal	Before	After	Notes
Saturday > > >	Breakfast			
	Lunch			
	Dinner			
	Bedtime			

Day	Meal	Before	After	Notes
Sunday > > >	Breakfast			
	Lunch			
	Dinner			
	Bedtime			

Weekly Blood Sugar Log

Week: ▓▓▓▓▓▓▓▓▓   Weight: ▓▓▓▓▓▓▓▓▓

Day	Meal	Before	After	Notes
Monday > > >	Breakfast			
	Lunch			
	Dinner			
	Bedtime			

Day	Meal	Before	After	Notes
Tuesday > > >	Breakfast			
	Lunch			
	Dinner			
	Bedtime			

Day	Meal	Before	After	Notes
Wednesday > > >	Breakfast			
	Lunch			
	Dinner			
	Bedtime			

Day	Meal	Before	After	Notes
Thursday > > >	Breakfast			
	Lunch			
	Dinner			
	Bedtime			

Day	Meal	Before	After	Notes
Friday > > >	Breakfast			
	Lunch			
	Dinner			
	Bedtime			

Day	Meal	Before	After	Notes
Saturday > > >	Breakfast			
	Lunch			
	Dinner			
	Bedtime			

Day	Meal	Before	After	Notes
Sunday > > >	Breakfast			
	Lunch			
	Dinner			
	Bedtime			

Weekly Blood Sugar Log

Week: _____   Weight: _____

Day	Meal	Before	After	Notes
Monday > > >	Breakfast			
	Lunch			
	Dinner			
	Bedtime			

Day	Meal	Before	After	Notes
Tuesday > > >	Breakfast			
	Lunch			
	Dinner			
	Bedtime			

Day	Meal	Before	After	Notes
Wednesday > > >	Breakfast			
	Lunch			
	Dinner			
	Bedtime			

Day	Meal	Before	After	Notes
Thursday > > >	Breakfast			
	Lunch			
	Dinner			
	Bedtime			

Day	Meal	Before	After	Notes
Friday > > >	Breakfast			
	Lunch			
	Dinner			
	Bedtime			

Day	Meal	Before	After	Notes
Saturday > > >	Breakfast			
	Lunch			
	Dinner			
	Bedtime			

Day	Meal	Before	After	Notes
Sunday > > >	Breakfast			
	Lunch			
	Dinner			
	Bedtime			

Weekly Blood Sugar Log

Week: _____   Weight: _____

Day	Meal	Before	After	Notes
Monday > > >	Breakfast			
	Lunch			
	Dinner			
	Bedtime			

Day	Meal	Before	After	Notes
Tuesday > > >	Breakfast			
	Lunch			
	Dinner			
	Bedtime			

Day	Meal	Before	After	Notes
Wednesday > > >	Breakfast			
	Lunch			
	Dinner			
	Bedtime			

Day	Meal	Before	After	Notes
Thursday > > >	Breakfast			
	Lunch			
	Dinner			
	Bedtime			

Day	Meal	Before	After	Notes
Friday > > >	Breakfast			
	Lunch			
	Dinner			
	Bedtime			

Day	Meal	Before	After	Notes
Saturday > > >	Breakfast			
	Lunch			
	Dinner			
	Bedtime			

Day	Meal	Before	After	Notes
Sunday > > >	Breakfast			
	Lunch			
	Dinner			
	Bedtime			

Weekly Blood Sugar Log

Week: _____   Weight: _____

Day	Meal	Before	After	Notes
Monday > > >	Breakfast			
	Lunch			
	Dinner			
	Bedtime			

Day	Meal	Before	After	Notes
Tuesday > > >	Breakfast			
	Lunch			
	Dinner			
	Bedtime			

Day	Meal	Before	After	Notes
Wednesday > > >	Breakfast			
	Lunch			
	Dinner			
	Bedtime			

Day	Meal	Before	After	Notes
Thursday > > >	Breakfast			
	Lunch			
	Dinner			
	Bedtime			

Day	Meal	Before	After	Notes
Friday > > >	Breakfast			
	Lunch			
	Dinner			
	Bedtime			

Day	Meal	Before	After	Notes
Saturday > > >	Breakfast			
	Lunch			
	Dinner			
	Bedtime			

Day	Meal	Before	After	Notes
Sunday > > >	Breakfast			
	Lunch			
	Dinner			
	Bedtime			

Weekly Blood Sugar Log

Week: _____   Weight: _____

Day	Meal	Before	After	Notes
Monday > > >	Breakfast			
	Lunch			
	Dinner			
	Bedtime			

Day	Meal	Before	After	Notes
Tuesday > > >	Breakfast			
	Lunch			
	Dinner			
	Bedtime			

Day	Meal	Before	After	Notes
Wednesday > > >	Breakfast			
	Lunch			
	Dinner			
	Bedtime			

Day	Meal	Before	After	Notes
Thursday > > >	Breakfast			
	Lunch			
	Dinner			
	Bedtime			

Day	Meal	Before	After	Notes
Friday > > >	Breakfast			
	Lunch			
	Dinner			
	Bedtime			

Day	Meal	Before	After	Notes
Saturday > > >	Breakfast			
	Lunch			
	Dinner			
	Bedtime			

Day	Meal	Before	After	Notes
Sunday > > >	Breakfast			
	Lunch			
	Dinner			
	Bedtime			

Weekly Blood Sugar Log

Week: _____   Weight: _____

Day	Meal	Before	After	Notes
Monday > > >	Breakfast			
	Lunch			
	Dinner			
	Bedtime			

Day	Meal	Before	After	Notes
Tuesday > > >	Breakfast			
	Lunch			
	Dinner			
	Bedtime			

Day	Meal	Before	After	Notes
Wednesday > > >	Breakfast			
	Lunch			
	Dinner			
	Bedtime			

Day	Meal	Before	After	Notes
Thursday > > >	Breakfast			
	Lunch			
	Dinner			
	Bedtime			

Day	Meal	Before	After	Notes
Friday > > >	Breakfast			
	Lunch			
	Dinner			
	Bedtime			

Day	Meal	Before	After	Notes
Saturday > > >	Breakfast			
	Lunch			
	Dinner			
	Bedtime			

Day	Meal	Before	After	Notes
Sunday > > >	Breakfast			
	Lunch			
	Dinner			
	Bedtime			

Notes

Notes

Notes

Notes